MIGRAINE DIET SMOOTHIES

Over 30 Delicious & Healthy Smoothies Based On The Migraine Diet Specifically Designed To Contain Beneficial Ingredients For Migraine Sufferers

By Michelle Strong

ISBN-13: 978-1530306084

ISBN-10: 1530306086

DISCLAIMER

CONTENTS

NUTRITION SNAPSHOT OF INGREDIENTS

In alphabetical order:

Apricots	5
Asparagus	5
Baby Spinach	5
Beetroot	5
Blackberries	6
Blueberries	6
Broccoli	6
Cantaloupe	7
Carrots	7
Celery	7
Cherries	8
Cilantro/Coriander	8
Coconut Flesh	8
Coconut Milk	9
Coconut Water	9
Cottage Cheese	9
Cucumbers	9
Dragonfruit	10
Flax seed	10
Ginger	10
Green Apples	10
Honey	10
Kale	11
Kiwi Fruit	11
Lemongrass	11

Michelle Strong

NUTRITIONAL ANALYSIS OF INGREDIENTS

Apricots

Apricots contain significant amounts of the vitamins A, C, K, E, as well as the minerals magnesium, potassium, manganese, copper, and phosphorous. Apricots are also a very good source of dietary fibre, with 2g per 100g.

Asparagus

Asparagus is very high in fibre, with 2.1g fibre per 100g. It is a rich source of vitamin B6, zinc, calcium and magnesium and very good source of vitamins C, E, K, beta-carotene (vitamin A), thiamine, riboflavin, rutin, niacin, folic acid, phosphorus, copper, selenium, iron, potassium, copper and manganese.

Baby Spinach

Baby spinach is high in vitamin A, vitamin K and folate. To increase the nutrients of spinach the body can absorb it has to be cooked. Cooking spinach will give you 600% more nutrition over eating it raw.

Beetroot

Beetroot contains Choline, a very important nutrient for migraine sufferers that has been widely reported to improve deep sleep and prevent insomnia, and prevent headaches. Choline also helps with reducing chronic inflammation. Beets contain betaine which is used in certain treatments of depression. They also contain tryptophan, which is a mind relaxant and gives a sense of well-being, as does chocolate. For migraine sufferers eating beets after a migraine could help with post migraine depression/hangover.

Blackberries

Blackberries have the highest content of antioxidants of any food, far above all others. The flavonoid that gives blackberries their deep colouring is a powerful phytonutrient that can protect the brain from oxidative stress. Consuming blackberries regularly may positively impact on health and reduce the effects of age-related conditions. They are also an extremely rich source of vitamin C and contain 5g fibre per 100g serving.

Blueberries

Blueberries are widely known as one of the superfoods. They contain anti-inflammatory and antibacterial properties, are rich in disease-fighting antioxidants, as well as B vitamins, fibre and vitamins C, E and K.

Broccoli

Broccoli is a rich source of fibre, both soluble and insoluble. It is an extremely rich source of vitamin C, with a 100g providing more than 150% of the recommended daily allowance. It is also a rich source of vitamins A, K, and B complex, iron, zinc, phosphorous and phyto-nutrients. It also has a high calcium content. Broccoli should be lightly cooked for 3-5 minutes to increase its health benefits as the body cannot process all the nutrients when it is raw.

Cantaloupe

Cantaloupe is extremely high in vitamin A, with 100g providing 112% of the recommended daily allowance. Protecting eye health is essential for migraine sufferers, as eye strain is a cause of migraines. Getting enough vitamin A in your diet is the first way to maintain eye health, as it assists eyes retain their ability to adjust to changes in light and maintains necessary eye moisture. It also helps to protect against age related macular degeneration. Cantaloupe is high in both fibre and water content, which helps to prevent constipation and promote a healthy digestive tract.

Carrots

Eye strain can be a cause of migraines, so maintaining optimal eye health should be a priority for migraine sufferers. Getting enough vitamin A, also known as retinol, in your diet is the first way to maintain eye health, as it assists eyes retain their ability to adjust to changes in light and maintains necessary moisture. It also helps to protect against age related macular degeneration. One medium sized carrot contains twice the daily recommended dose of vitamin A. Carrots are also a good source of vitamins C and K, and potassium.

Celery

Celery reduces inflammation, great for migraine sufferers whose migraines are caused by arthritis in the neck. The minerals in celery, especially magnesium, make it great for stress relief, another migraine trigger. Due to its high water content and insoluble fibre it is a great digestive aid and remedy for constipation, another migraine trigger. It also is a good source of calcium and vitamin B2.

Cherries

Cherries are great for migraine sufferers. Not only do they have a very high water content at 75%, and are high in fibre at nearly 3g a serving, but they are also very high in the anti-oxidant melatonin which soothes brain neurons, which calms nervous system irritability. Nervous system irritability can directly cause migraines and insomnia, so this is an important nutrient to include in your diet.

Cilantro/Coriander

One-quarter cup of cilantro is extremely high in vitamin K, the riches herbal plant source of this vitamin. It is a rich source of many vitamins including the B group vitamins, vitamin C, and vitamin A.

Coconut Flesh

Coconut flesh is extremely high in the mineral manganese, one cup providing 67% of the recommended daily allowance. Manganese is a vital mineral for migraine sufferers. it helps metabolize both fat and protein, supports the nervous system and promotes stable blood sugar levels. Coconut flesh is also extremely high in fibre, one cup containing 7.2g of fibre, more than 20 percent of the recommended daily amount.

Coconut Milk

As most migraine sufferers should avoid dairy products, coconut milk can be used as a delicious substitute for milk, although it is much higher in calories so a careful watch should be kept on daily intake. It is rich in fibre, one cup providing 5g, and vitamins C, E, B1, B3, B5 and B6. It also contains minerals such as iron, magnesium, sodium, selenium, calcium, and phosphorous.

Coconut Water

Coconut water is composed of many naturally occurring bioactive enzymes which help with digestion and metabolism. It has a better composition than some fruit juices of minerals such as manganese, calcium, magnesium, iron, and zinc. It is a very good source of B group vitamins and potassium.

Cottage Cheese

Cottage cheese contains a large amount of calcium, a mineral necessary for vascular function which is important for migraine sufferers as studies have indicated they are at increased risk of vascular disease. It is also a complete protein in itself, and contains phosphorous, potassium, folate, vitamin A and zinc.

Cucumbers

Cucumbers are from the same family as melons. They contain a high water content of 96%. For migraine sufferers, dehydration is one of the most common causes of a migraine. The vitamins cucumbers contain include high levels of vitamin C, which is important for brain function and lowering the risk of cancers and illness; and vitamin K, half of which is found its skin, so if you have a high-speed blender you could leave the skin on.

Dragonfruit

Dragon fruit is rich in vitamin C, B1, B2 and B3, and minerals such as iron, calcium, and phosphorus.

Flax seed

Flax seed is one of the superfoods. It contains 50-60% of omega-3 fatty acids, is extremely high in both soluble and insoluble fibre, and is high in most of the B vitamins, manganese and magnesium.

Ginger

Ginger is great for migraine sufferers. It is aids digestion, relieves nausea, and is an anti-inflammatory.

Green Apples

Red apples are a known migraine trigger. Luckily, green apples are healthier for you. They contain less sugar, more fibre, higher antioxidant levels, and more vitamins. They are great for stabilizing blood sugar, and contain carbohydrates which are good for energy, as well as being high in protein.

Honey

Honey stabilizes blood sugar which is vital for migraine sufferers. A drop in blood sugar levels can be a trigger for migraines. It gives an immediate energy boost by absorbing glucose quickly, while providing sustained energy by absorbing fructose more slowly.

Kale

Currently sitting at the top of the ladder of the superfoods is kale. One cup of raw kale contains 3g of protein, 2.5g fibre, vitamins A,C and K, folate, omega-3 fatty acids, nutrients that protect against cataracts and macular degeneration, and minerals iron, copper, potassium, manganese, phosphorous, zinc, calcium and potassium. When cooked, kale has 1000% more vitamin C than cooked spinach, and is better absorbed by the body than spinach.

Kiwi Fruit

Kiwi fruit is extremely high in vitamin C, one cup providing 270% of the daily allowance. It is also extremely high in vitamin K, with one cup providing 89% of the recommended daily allowance. It has more potassium than a banana, and extremely high in fibre.

Lemongrass

Lemongrass is used in tea to treat digestive problems such as spasms, pain, vomiting, stomach ache, achy joints, and exhaustion, so is a good herb for migraine sufferers. It is extremely high in iron, one tablespoon containing 4mg, which is 5% of the recommended daily intake.

Lettuce Iceberg

Lettuce is very high in dietary fibre, iron, magnesium, potassium, vitamin A, B6, C, and high in calcium and vitamin E.

Lettuce - Romaine/Cos

Romaine lettuce is a good source of vitamin C, providing 10% more than iceberg lettuce. It is high in fibre, rich in vitamin A and folate. It is a good source of iron, calcium and potassium.

Mango

Less than one cup of ripe mango provides up to three times the recommended daily intake of vitamins A and C. They are also a rich source of beta-carotene, fibre and potassium.

Melon

Dehydration is one of the major triggers of migraines so keeping hydrated is vitally important for migraine sufferers. Melons and cucumbers are from the same family and both contain a high water content of 95%. This also promotes good digestion and avoids constipation. Melons good for an energy boost as they contain the B group vitamins which are responsible for the body's energy production in processing sugar and carbohydrates. Cucumbers have high levels of vitamin C, which is important for brain function and lowering the risk of cancers and illness; and vitamin K, half of which is found its skin.

Mint

Mint soothes stomach indigestion or inflammation and promotes digestion. It is very effective for nausea, even just by smelling it.

Nectarines

Nectarines are very similar to peaches but they contain many more minerals and vitamins. They contain double the amount of vitamins A and C, and also contain vitamins B1, B2, B3, B6, E, K and folate. They are a great source of potassium, phosphorous, calcium and magnesium. The skin of nectarines contains most of its antioxidants so leave it on to eat it, just was it first.

Oats

Oats are extremely high in fibre, one cup providing half the daily recommended intake. As a result they are very effective at stabilising blood sugar levels, which is very important for migraine sufferers. They contain the minerals selenium, manganese, phosphorus, zinc and magnesium.

Parsley

Parsley contains high amounts of vitamins A, C and K, and helps the body absorb iron and vitamin K from other foods. It is rich in antioxidants and is a good source of calcium, potassium, magnesium and manganese.

Peaches

A peach contains 10 different kinds of vitamins: A, C, E, K and six of the B complex vitamins. Peaches are also a source of thiamine, riboflavin, vitamin B-6, niacin, folate, and pantothenic acid, all valuable nutrients when it comes to your cells and nerves.

Pears

Pears are one of the best sources of dietary fibre, with 8% of fibre per 100g fruit. They are a good source of vitamins C, E, B2, copper and potassium.

Pearl Barley

Pearl Barley is one of the recommended foods for migraine sufferers. It is extremely high in fibre, with 6 grams per cup, and an excellent source of several B vitamins and good amounts of most of the B group vitamins. Pearl Barley is also high in Selenium, a trace mineral which supports the immune system.

Pomegranate seeds

Pomegranate seeds are high in fibre, with 1/2 cup providing 3.5g, and a good source of vitamins, C and K. A 100g serving contains 10.2 mg of vitamin C (17% of the recommended daily allowance) and 16mcg of vitamin K (20% of the recommended daily allowance.

Pumpkin

Pumpkin is extremely high in vitamin A, with 100g providing 246% of the recommended daily allowance. It is also a rich source of vitamins C and E, rich in dietary fibre, antioxidants and minerals copper, calcium potassium and phosphorus.

Quinoa

Coming second on the superfood ladder would have to be quinoa (pronounced keen-wah). This is a great food for migraine sufferers, as it contains magnesium, manganese, phosphorous and folate. Magnesium is a key nutrient for migraine sufferers and for the body to absorb it optimally it needs adequate amounts of vitamin B6, which quinoa also contains. Quinoa, although a plant food, is a complete protein. One quarter of a cup provides 6g of protein, as well as 27g carbohydrates, but no cholesterol or sodium.

Red Cabbage

Raw red cabbage contains significant amounts of vitamins C, K, A, B6 and folate. It also contains the minerals manganese, iron, calcium, zine and phosphorous. Red cabbage contains one of the highest levels of antioxidants of all vegetables - 36 different flavonoids, which means for migraine sufferers an improvement in neurological function.

Strawberries

Strawberries are a good anti-inflammatory as they contain phytonutrients and are an antioxidant. Importantly they are a rich source of fibre, folate, vitamin C, and B-vitamins. As an antioxidant they are good for their anti-cancer properties as well.

Soy Milk

Migraine sufferers should avoid all processed soy products as they are a known migraine trigger, unless through the elimination diet they have proven to not be one of your triggers. Soy milk, however, should be safe as it is not processed. It is beneficial in the diet as adding soy to the diet is known to prevent prostate cancer in men and improve post-menopausal symptoms in women.

Starfruit

Starfruit is an excellent source of fibre, is rich in vitamin C and a good source of vitamin A. It contains the minerals magnesium, which is especially good for migraine sufferers, and is rich in copper. It contains a large amount of antioxidants, of the type found in red wine, chocolate and green tea. It also contains choline, a very important nutrient for migraine sufferers that has been widely reported to improve deep sleep and prevent insomnia, and prevent headaches.

Swiss Chard

Swiss Chard/Silverbeet is an excellent source of vitamins A, C, K, omega-3 fatty acids, B complex vitamins and a rich source of minerals such as iron, copper, calcium, sodium, manganese, potassium and phosphorus. It regulates blood sugar levels, aids in the prevention of various types of cancer, improves digestion, boosts the immune system, reduces fever and combats inflammation, lowers blood pressure, prevents heart disease, increases bone strength and development, detoxifies the body, and strengthens the functioning of the brain.

Watermelon

Watermelon is a good source of potassium and magnesium. Potassium is a vasodilator, ie it releases the tension of blood vessels and arteries, and stimulates increased blood flow which is beneficial for migraine attacks. It is also extremely high in water content, aiding in digestion and averting constipation.

Michelle Strong

SMOOTHIES

Rehydrating Melon-Cucumber Smo

Serves: 2

Preparation Time: 10 minutes

Ingredients:

2 cups melon cubes

1/2 cucumber, peeled

2 cups coconut water

2 tsp natural honey, optional

Directions:

Add coconut water and cucumber into a high-speed blender.
Blend until smooth.

Add melon and honey and blend well.

Serve and enjoy!

Nutritional information per serving:

Calories: 135
Carbs: 31 g,
Fats: 0.8 g
Protein: 3 g

Two Layer Smoothie

Serves: 2

Preparation Time: 10 minutes

Ingredients:

1/2 cup beets, cooked and peeled

½ cup strawberries, frozen

½ cup green apple

½ cup celery

2 tsp natural honey

2 cups coconut water

Directions:

Place the beets, strawberries, 1 tsp honey and 1 cup coconut water in a blender and blend on high speed until smooth and thick.

Pour in a tall glass.

Place the apple, celery and rest of honey and coconut water in the blender and puree.

Pour on top of the strawberry-beet smoothie.

Nutritional information per serving:

Calories: 111

Carbs: 25.3g

Fats: 7.2g

Protein: 2.8g

Green Mint & Cucumber Migraine Re
Smoothie

Serves: 2

Preparation Time: 10 minutes,

Ingredients:

2 cucumbers, peeled and roughly chopped

¼ cup fresh mint leaves

1 green apple

1 cup mint tea, cold

2 cups coconut water

2 tsp natural honey

1 cup ice

Directions:

Place all the ingredients in a high speed blender and puree.

Pour in a tall glass.

Garnish with fresh mint leaves

Serve and enjoy.

Nutritional information per serving:

Calories: 130
Carbs: 29 g
Fats: 0.9 g
Protein: 3.1 g

Very Berry Smoothie

Serves: 2

Preparation Time: 10 minutes

Ingredients:

½ cup low fat cottage cheese

1 cup blackberries

1 cup blueberries

¼ tsp vanilla extract

2 cups coconut water

Directions:

Place all the ingredients in a high speed processor and blend well.

Pour in a tall glass and serve

Nutritional information per serving:

Calories: 159
Carbs: 28.1
Fats: 1.6g
Protein: 10.3g

Simply Detoxing Smoothie

Serves: 2

Preparation Time: 10 minutes

Ingredients:

2 pears, seeds removed

½ cup baby spinach, cooked

2 tbsp fresh parsley, chopped

2 cups coconut water

Directions:

Place all the ingredients in a blender, blend on high speed until smooth and thick.

Pour in tall glasses.

Garnish with fresh strawberries.

Serve.

Nutritional information per serving:

Calories: 140
Carbs: 33.1g
Fats: 0.8g
Protein: 3.6g

Green Barley Smoothie

Serves: 2

Preparation Time: 10 minutes

Ingredients:

¼ cup uncooked pearl barley

1 cup Swiss chard/Silverbeet

1 peach, stone removed

2 cups coconut milk

2 tsp natural honey, optional

Directions:

Bring 1 cup of water to a boil; add the barley and cook until fluffy or until all water is absorbed.

Place all the ingredients into a high-speed blender, liquids first, and blend well until smooth.

Serve.

Nutritional information per serving:

Calories: 185
Carbs: 42 g
Fats: 1.0g
Protein: 5.25g

Superfood Cranberry Smoothie w Ginger

Serves: 2

Preparation Time: 10 minutes

Ingredients:

1.5 cup cranberries, frozen

1 tsp grated ginger

1 cup coconut milk

1 cup filtered water

2 tsp natural honey, optional

Directions:

Add all the ingredients into a high-speed blender, liquids first.

Blend well until smooth.

Serve.

Nutritional information per serving:

Calories: 335

Carbs: 22.5g

Fats: 28.7g

Protein: 3.1g

Spicy Apple Smoothie

Serves: 2

Preparation Time: 10 minutes

Ingredients:

2 carrots, peeled and roughly chopped

2 green apples, peeled and roughly chopped

2 cups filtered water

½ cup crushed ice

1 tbsp natural honey

Directions:

Place all the ingredients – except ice - in a high speed processor and blend well until all ingredients are combined.

Pour in a tall glass.

Top with crushed ice.

Serve and enjoy!

Nutritional information per serving:

Calories: 134
Carbs: 35g
Fats: 0.4g
Protein: 1.0g

Celery Smoothie

Serves: 2

Preparation Time: 10 minutes

Ingredients:

1 cup celery, cooked

½ cup baby spinach, cooked

2 tsp flaxseeds

2 tsp natural honey

1 cup coconut milk

1 cup filtered water

Directions:

Place all the ingredients in a high speed processor, liquids first, and blend well.

Pour in a short glass, garnish with celery sticks and serve!

Nutritional information per serving:

Calories: 312
Carbs: 10.8g
Fats: 30.2g
Protein: 5g

Summer Breeze Smoothie

Preparation Time: 10 minutes

Ingredients:

2 cups watermelon cubes

1 cup frozen strawberries (Blueberries / blackberries)

1 cup coconut water

Directions:

Add coconut water and watermelon into a high-speed blender.

Blend until smooth.

Add the rest of ingredients and blend well.

Serve and enjoy!

Nutritional information per serving:

Calories: 92.5

Carbs: 21.7g

Fats: 0.7g

Protein: 2.3g

Detoxing Vegan Smoothie

Serves: 2

Preparation Time: 10 minutes

Ingredients:

2 kiwis, peeled and sliced

1 cup lettuce

2 tbsp fresh cilantro/coriander

2 cups coconut water

¼ cup crushed ice

Directions:

Place all the ingredients in a blender and blend on high speed.

Pour in a tall glass, top with crushed ice and garnish with fresh kiwi slices.

Serve and enjoy!

Nutritional information per serving:

Calories: 90
Carbs: 19.3g
Fats: 7.5g
Protein: 2.7g

Three-Colour Smoothie

Time: 15 minutes

Ingredients:

½ cup blueberries, frozen

½ cup strawberries, frozen (blackberry)

1 green apple deseeded and roughly chopped

½ cup coconut cream

1 cup filtered water

Directions:

Add ½ cup water and strawberries into a blender

Blend well and pour in a large glass (covering the 1/3 of the glass)

Add coconut milk and apple into a blender

Blend well and pour on top of the strawberry smoothie.

Add ½ cup water and blueberries into a blender.

Blend well and carefully pour on top of the strawberry/apple smoothie.

Garnish with fresh blueberries, serve and enjoy!

Nutritional information per serving:

Calories: 229
Carbs: 40g
Fats: 8.3g
Protein: 1.1g

Tropical Splash Smoothie

Serves: 2

Preparation Time: 10 minutes

Ingredients:

1 cup mango chunks

½ cup coconut chunks

1 cup coconut milk

1 cup coconut water

2 tsp brown sugar, optional

Directions:

Add all the ingredients into a blender, liquids first.

Blend until smooth and thick.

Serve in a tall glass and enjoy!

Nutritional information per serving:

Calories: 407
Carbs: 25g
Fats: 35.6g
Protein: 4.1g

Migraine Beet & Blueberry Smoothie

Serves: 2

Preparation Time: 10 minutes

Ingredients:

1/2 cup beets, cooked and peeled

1 cup frozen blueberries

2 cups coconut water

2 tsp maple syrup, optional

Directions:

Add coconut water and beets into a high-speed blender.

Blend well.

Add blueberries and blend.

Pour in tall glass.

Serve and enjoy!

Nutritional information per serving:

Calories: 129

Carbs: 29.6g

Fats: 0.8g

Protein: 2.8g

Apple, Mint & Lemon Grass Smoothie

Serves: 2

Preparation Time: 10 minutes

Ingredients:

2 green apples, seeds removed and roughly chopped

¼ cup lemongrass

2 tbsp fresh mint

1 cup coconut milk

1 cup coconut water

Directions:

Place all the ingredients in a high speed processor and blend well.

Pour in a tall glass and serve.

Nutritional information per serving:

Calories: 378
Carbs: 33.9g
Fats: 28.9g
Protein: 3.4g

Cantaloupe Smoothie

Serves: 2

Preparation Time: 10 minutes

Ingredients:

2 cups cantaloupe melon

1 green apple, deseeded and roughly chopped

½ tsp vanilla extract

¼ tsp nutmeg

¼ tsp cinnamon

2 cups filtered water

Directions:

Place all the ingredients in a high speed processor and blend well.

Pour in a tall glass and serve

Nutritional information per serving:

Calories: 93

Carbs: 23.3g

Fats: 0.4g

Protein: 1.5g

Pumpkin Spice Smoothie

Serves: 2

Preparation Time: 10 minutes

Ingredients:

1 cup pumpkin

1 green apple, peeled and roughly chopped

¼ tsp anise seeds

¼ tsp cinnamon

1 cup coconut milk

1 cup filtered water

2 tsp maple syrup, optional

Directions:

Bring 2 cups of water to a boil and cook the pumpkin for about 20 minutes or until soft.

Add all the ingredients in a blender and mix well.

Nutritional information per serving:

Calories: 339

Carbs: 23.3g

Fats: 28.7g

Protein: 2.7g

Pink Love Smoothie

Serves: 2

Preparation Time: 10 minutes

Ingredients:

1 cup red dragon fruit

1 cup blackberries

1 cup coconut milk

1 cup filtered water

Fresh mint to garnish

Directions:

Place all the ingredients in a blender, liquids first, and blend on high speed until really smooth.

Pour in a white wine-type tumbler glass, garnish with fresh mint and serve.

Nutritional information per serving:

Calories: 326

Carbs: 19.7g

Fats: 26.6g

Protein: 2.0g

Garden Vegetable Smoothie

Serves: 2

Preparation Time: 10 minute

Ingredients:

1 cup baby spinach, cooked

½ cup broccoli, cooked lightly

½ cup kale

1 cup coconut milk

1 cup filtered water

2 tbsp maple syrup

Directions:

Place all the ingredients in a blender, liquids first and blend on high speed until smooth.

Pour in large, tall glasses.

Serve.

Nutritional information per serving:

Calories: 322.4

Carbs: 16.9g

Fats: 28.9g

Protein: 4.5g

Green Starfruit Smoothie

Serves: 2

Preparation Time: 10 minute

Ingredients:

1 cup star fruit, sliced

1 cup kiwi, sliced

2 tbsp fresh mint

1 tbsp chia seeds

2 cups coconut water

Directions:

Place all the ingredients in a blender, liquids first and chia seeds last, and blend well.

Pour into a short glass.

Serve with ice.

Enjoy!

Nutritional information per serving:

Calories: 147
Carbs: 8.9g
Fats: 3.0g
Protein: 1.7g

Blueberry Indulgence Smoothie

Serves: 2

Preparation Time: 15 minutes

Ingredients:

1 cup frozen blueberries

½ cup frozen cranberries

2 tsp flaxseeds

2 cups filtered water

1 tbsp natural honey (optional)

Directions:

Place all the ingredients in a high speed blender and blend very well.

Pour in short glasses.

Serve and enjoy!

Nutritional information per serving:

Calories: 118.5

Carbs: 27.2g

Fats: 1.7g

Protein: 1.4g

The Low Calorie Smoothie

Serves: 2

Preparation Time: 10 minutes

Ingredients:

1 cup frozen blackberries

½ cup red cabbage

2 cups filtered water

2 tsp natural honey

1 cup ice

Directions:

Place all the ingredients in a blender and blend on high speed until smooth and thick.

Pour in a tall glass.

Enjoy!

Nutritional information per serving:

Calories: 59
Carbs: 14.4g
Fats: 0.4g
Protein: 1.3g

Green Apple Smoothie

Serves: 2

Preparation Time: 70 minutes

Ingredients:

2 green apples, seeds removed and roughly chopped

2 apricots, stones removed

½ cup coconut cream

2 cups filtered water

Directions:

Freeze apples for at least an hour.

Place all the ingredients in a blender and blend on high speed until smooth and thick.

Pour in a tall glass, and serve.

Nutritional information per serving:

Calories: 77

Carbs: 63.5g

Fats: 12.4g

Protein: 1.8g

Rainbow Smoothie

Serves: 2

Preparation Time: 10 minutes

Ingredients:

½ cup blueberries, frozen

½ cup coconut chunks

½ cup cranberries, frozen

2 cups coconut water

Directions:

Place the blueberries and ½ cup water into a high speed food processor and blend well.

Pour in a tall glass.

Place the coconut and ½ cup water in the processor and puree.

Pour on top of blueberries.

Repeat with strawberries and rest of water.

Serve and enjoy!

Nutritional information per serving:

Calories: 150

Carbs: 20.6g

Fats: 7.3g

Protein: 1.7g

The Vitamin Booster Smoothie

Serves: 2

Preparation Time: 10 minutes

Ingredients:

1 cup romaine/cos lettuce

¼ cup cooked asparagus

2 apricots

2 cups unsweetened soy milk

2 tsp maple syrup or molasses

Ice

Directions:

Place all the ingredients in a blender, liquids first, and blend until smooth and thick.

Serve over ice.

Nutritional information per serving:

Calories: 85.5

Carbs: 4.4g

Fats: 1.0g

Protein: 2.8g

Dragon Fruit & Pomegranate Smoothie

Serves: 2

Preparation Time: 10 minutes

Ingredients:

1 cup dragon fruit chunks

1 cup pomegranate seeds

2 tbsp fresh mint

1 cup coconut milk

1 cup filtered water

Directions:

Place the dragon fruit chinks and pomegranate seeds into a high speed blender and puree.

Add the liquids and blend again.

Garnish with fresh mint.

Serve in a tall glass together with ice.

Nutritional information per serving:

Calories: 376
Carbs: 30.4g
Fats: 29.7g
Protein: 4.3g

Strawberry & Coconut Swirl

Serves: 2

Preparation Time: 10 minutes

Ingredients:

1 green apple, seeds and skin removed, roughly chopped

½ cup frozen strawberries

½ cup coconut chunks

1 cup coconut milk

1 cup filtered water

Directions:

Place the strawberries and water in a blender and puree.

Pour in a highball glass.

Place the coconut, coconut milk and apple in the blender and puree.

Slowly pour the coconut mixture into the centre of the pureed strawberries in order to form swirls.

Nutritional information per serving:

Calories: 430

Carbs: 31.5g

Fats: 35.5g

Protein: 4.0g

Super Healthy Quinoa Smoothie

Serves: 3
Preparation Time: 10 minutes

Ingredients:

½ cup cooked quinoa

2 apricots, stones removed

1 cup coconut chunks

4-5 cherries

2.5 cup filtered water

Directions:

Place the quinoa and coconut in a blender and puree.

Add the rest of ingredients and blend well.

Pour in a cocktail glass.

Garnish with cherries and serve!

Nutritional information per serving:

Calories: 308
Carbs: 14.3g
Fats: 28.4g
Protein: 3.7g

Simply Delicious Peach Smoothie

Serves: 3

Preparation Time: 10 minutes

Ingredients:

2 medium sized peaches, stones removed and roughly chopped

2 medium sized nectarines, stones removed and roughly chopped

3 cups coconut water

½ tsp vanilla extract

Directions:

Add all the ingredients in a high speed blender, liquids first.

Puree.

Pour in a tumbler glass.

Serve and enjoy!

Nutritional information per serving:

Calories: 126
Carbs: 42.6g
Fats: 1.0g
Protein: 3.6g

Healthy Broccoli Smoothie

Serves: 3

Preparation Time: 10 minutes

Ingredients:

1 cup broccoli florets, cooked lightly

2 green apples, seeds removed and roughly chopped

2 tsp fresh mint

2 cups coconut water

2 tsp maple syrup

Directions:

Place all the ingredients in a high speed processor and blend well.

Pour in a tall glass and serve.

Nutritional information per serving:

Calories: 107.6

Carbs: 35.9g

Fats: 0.9g

Protein: 3.6g

Red Velvet Smoothie

Serves: 2

Preparation Time: 10 minutes

Ingredients:

1 cup fresh cherries, seeds removed

1 cup frozen strawberries

1 cup coconut milk

1 cup filtered water

1 tbsp natural honey

Directions:

Place all the ingredients in a high speed processor and blend well.

Pour in a tall glass and serve.

Nutritional information per serving:

Calories: 383
Carbs: 34.1g
Fats: 29.0g
Protein: 4.1g

Simply Delicious 2-layer Smoothie

Serves: 2

Preparation Time: 10 minutes

Ingredients:

8 tbsp oats

½ cup frozen strawberries

3-4 apricots, seeds removed

2 cups coconut milk

Directions:

Place the strawberries and 1 cup of coconut milk in a blender and puree.

Pour in a tall glass (approximately ½ of the glass).

Place the apricots, oats and 1 cup of coconut milk in a blender and puree.

Pour on top of the strawberry smoothie.

Nutritional information per serving:

Calories: 552

Carbs: 50.3g

Fats: 60.2g

Protein: 13.4g

Sweet Nectarine Smoothie

Serves: 2

Preparation Time: 10 minutes

Ingredients:

2 nectarines, stones removed

½ cup melon

1 carrot, thinly sliced

1 cup coconut milk

1 cup coconut water

Directions:

Place all the ingredients in a blender and blend on high speed until smooth and thick.

Pour in large, tall glass.

Serve and enjoy!

Nutritional information per serving:

Calories: 365
Carbs: 28g
Fats: 29.1g
Protein: 4.9g

Suffering from regular migraines and trying to avoid your triggers at meal times?

The Migraine Diet Cookbook contains over 50 recipes without common migraine triggers or additives.

Based on the Headache Elimination Diet, this cookbook provides recipes that either don't contain the common migraine triggers, or have had them replaced with a non-trigger substitute. Many recipes include ingredients that contain nutrients that are known to be beneficial for migraine sufferers.

Plus detailed substitutes for common ingredients that are known migraine triggers.

This is more than just a cookbook, it's a reference that allows you to eliminate the common food and additive triggers from your diet every day so <u>YOU</u> control your migraines, instead of your migraines controlling you!

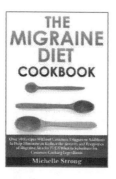

OTHER BOOKS BY SCG PUBLISHING

Keto Make Ahead Freezer Meals and Snacks by Skye Howard Registered & Licenced Dietician

Keto Smoothies & Shakes by Skye Howard RDLD

Keto One Pot Meals by Skye Howard RDLD

HIIT: High Intensity Interval Training - Look Like An Athlete Feel Like An Athlete by Steve Ryan BScExercise&NutritionBScSport

Chilli Jam Recipes by Amanda Kent

40753561R00039

Made in the USA
Middletown, DE
22 February 2017